Billie R. Tadros's *Graft Fixation* is fascinated by what comes together after a break—it's never quite the old form, but it's not fully a new one, either. The poems work around a car crash and subsequent injury in scattered, piecemeal forms, mirroring the way trauma isn't digested all at once or in a simple, understandable manner. The speaker knows they will never be who they used to be, but they seek a new agency, a fresh way to conceive of their identity in relation to and transcending the body. These poems are frantic and jagged, but they move towards an evolution.

— **Ruth Baumann, author of *Thornwork***

Graft Fixation takes apart the legal and medical language surrounding injury in a car crash, turns those words over and over, and reassembles this multi-layered language with a mixture of angry grief and intense playfulness. The resulting poems interrogate our understanding of bodies, especially women's bodies, through collisions of language and form: human/auto body, sexual/moving violation, good/bad pain. No description of this book could prepare you. Read it, and let it take you apart.

— **Katie Manning, author of *Tasty Other***

Graft Fixation is intense and powerful, truly a "cyborg" of medical and emotional language. You can feel the weight of the physical injury, the cold finality of the medical documents, the crushing blow of losing something you love. There are two stories here: the first is the cold, definitive medical truth; and the other is the raw, heart-breaking, uncertain truth of what life turns into now.

— **Rachael Steil, author of *Running in Silence: My Drive for Perfection and the Eating Disorder That Fed It***

D1596652

GRAFT FIXATION

BILLIE R. TADROS

Billie R. Tadros

GOLD WAKE

For all of the men who have entered my body
with my consent—

most of whom have been orthopedic surgeons.

The patient understood her diagnoses.

She was an avid runner.

—Operative Report ITS, 25 Jul. 2014

MVA Documentation — Mechanism of Injury

Drivers [*sic*] Name ██████████

Forces involved High
(Speed greater than 40 mph)

Mechanism of Injury Deformity greater
than 18 inches in vehicle

<u>Narrative History Text:</u>
THIS PATIENT WAS THE FRONT SEAT PASSENGER OF A SMALL SPORTS CAR THAT HAD A SIGNIFICANT FRONTAL IMPACT. SHE DID NOT LOSE CONSCIOUSNESS. SHE WAS RESTRAINED, HER AIRBAG DEPLOYED, AND SHE HAD NO COMPLAINTS. SHE APPEARED ATRAUMATIC AND I FOUND NO OBVIOUS INJURIES ON EXAM.

—Prehospital Care Summary, 6 May 2014

(There is always another version of this story.)

CONTENTS

Author's Note on Process

I composed some of the poems in this manuscript in part by performing erasures on source texts that detail a motor vehicle accident in which I was a passenger and on other source texts that address the legal and medical consequences of this accident—e.g., the police's accident report, medical reports from my emergency room visit and later medical visits, correspondence with insurance agents representing the defendant in my bodily injury claim, and medical pamphlets given to me by my surgeons.

I generated text for many of the other poems in this manuscript using the "What Would I Say?" Facebook app (www.what-would-i-say.com), which was created by seven Princeton graduate students in 2013. The app uses a Markov bot to produce text representing Facebook status updates from the archive of the user's previously posted Facebook status updates. Because I occasionally quoted other authors' texts in my Facebook status updates, phrases in some of the poems in *Graft Fixation* that developed from this compositional method sample these authors' texts. I credit these authors and their texts in my notes and references.

TO ENABLE US TO DETEMINE [*sic*] IF YOU ARE ENTITLED

TO BENEFITS UNDER THE PERSONAL INJURY PROTECTION LAW YOU MUST <u>COMPLETE</u> AND <u>SIGN</u> THIS FORM.

YOU MUST ALSO <u>SIGN</u> THE ATTACHED AUTHORIZATION(S).

RETURN PROMPTLY WITH ANY MEDICAL BILLS YOU HAVE RECEIVED TO DATE.

Do you or any member of your household own an automobile?	☒ YES ☐ NO
Were you the driver of the automobile?	☐ YES ☒ NO
Were you a passenger in the automobile?	☒ YES ☐ NO
As a result of this accident, were you injured?	☒ YES ☐ NO

On Miscalculating the Distance between Pardon and Forgiveness

Men always tell me what would prefer to speak
through pain. I learned from the starting line:

you have to decide if you move on.

I

Accident Report as Homophonic Translation

The passenger stated she was facing west. The driver's face
was in the wheel, or the driver's face was in the well

of his passenger's body. Or the car was a well.
The driver stated he was unable to avoid impact.

When the investigating officer arrived on scene
it was asphalt

and he said *Well*. (The passenger said that she was well
or the passenger said that she *was* a well. She was emptied.)

The emergency medical technician emptied the passenger
from the well of the car and said that she was well.

When the investigating officer arrived on scene
it was as fault.

Upon initial contact with the driver, the investigating
officer noted an odor of alcohol emitting from his person

and asked him to step out.

The driver said he was thirsty. The woman was no longer
his passenger. (She emitted that she was not his person.)

The driver said he couldn't stop—the vehicle. He admitted
that she was not his person. The driver said he couldn't

negotiate—the turn. The passenger was transported
by ambulance. (She would not walk.) The treating

physician's report said that she was well.

The road was a wound that swelled
around what was left—the vehicle.

The driver was turning left into the intersection.

(The driver turned their bodies into an intersection.)

The investigating officer reported that the passenger stated she was well:

She was restrained, and she had no complaints. She was no longer a passenger. She was admitted. She was

a road or a well or a wound. A well ridden wound.

The Ways I Had Known My Body Were a Few

fronds hanging from a femur.

He said *rapture*, I said
rupture. He said *collision*

I said *collusion*.

He said *faster*. I said *fast*.
He swerved.

I starved.

When I hit the curb I remembered the taste

of the smell of a smell, a meta-
olfaction, the sweet

exhaust and the spider
glass, how the windshield

webbed and caught me, its prey

or its salvage.

Surgery is a kind of elegy, its probes
and probity, its capillary truths.

Mechanism of Injury

Extent of deformity:
severe.[1] The passenger's skin

hit the wheel.[2] The passenger
said that she was well. She was

restrained, and she had no complaints.

The doctor noted a welt on the passenger.[3]

The driver said that she welled
her consent. Later she said that

he willed her. Later she called it

an accident.[4]

(The mechanic looked at the bumper and said *Weld.*[5])

---

[1] Here it's unclear whether we are narrativizing the body of the car or the body of the passenger.
[2] Who *wheeled*, who *wealed.* Who wielded.
[3] Accident rapport: deformity severe. (Wound or watermark.)
[4] *Accident* absolves, as in *The passenger said that she was well.* As in *She had no complaints.*
[5] Auto body. (Ought a body be well enough.)

Cannibalizing Two Broken-down Cars Might Provide Spare Parts to Make One Working Car

When I ask her to define *forgiveness*, my therapist
suggests that I write you a letter. But I neither want to

forgive you nor to *give* you anything else. (My knee
gives.) The epistolary, after all, is all about response

or the absence of response. After my first

surgery, when the numbness of the skin surrounding
the surgical site became sensate again, I learned

that there was something

erogenous about my response
to the touch of that scar

tissue that marked where part
of my patella had been harvested

and repurposed.

Hymen after Significant Frontal Impact

Last night and error, the smell
of scarred tissue when I sleep and pretending

this is when I fell the second time.

In fact it is a crucial boundary between
fiction and endurance.[1] The former feels

the ache[2] and the pockets are fantastic.

I can't keep finishing[3]
the floor with allografts.

---

[1] When I knew him—the man who later plied me with whiskey, coerced me into his vehicle, and then crashed that vehicle into the back of another vehicle—he would coyly introduce his work with the claim that everything he wrote was nonfiction "because it happened to [him]."

[2] There's evidence to suggest that women runners can differentiate between "good pain" and "bad pain" (see, for example, Hanold 172). Such a differentiation might colloquially be called "listening to [one's] body." Some women runners experience a great tension between their desire to "push through [bad] pain" and their understanding of what their bodies are "telling" them (see, for example, Tadros 126-127). But *desire* is not *consent.*

[3] This isn't a letter. Even nonfiction is fictive. (And it didn't happen to him.)

Automotive Body Cavity

My teeth hurt, I'm finding it very difficult to place
my mouth.

I suppose that's your depression grinding.

I can call my doctor and make some sounds
like coming—

In other words, everything is normal.

(Normalized.) If you're wondering
if it's endemic—I trusted you—

Localized.

The Anniversary Effect, Which Is Sometimes Called an Anniversary Reaction

This is the thanks—*I can't
remember,*[1] can't articulate the condyle.

It's sad, as always, to decide
if I trusted my body. I believed

in pain so I trusted that. I have to
acknowledge the boundary is important.

That was years ago, and for the week
I would like you on me as ice.

But then I would have to acknowledge
that I willed this. All I do know: I had not

already come to my body.

---

[1] *Had you been drinking?*

Underinsured Motorist Coverage

Dear Ms.,

As per our conversation, the referenced claim does not have applicable coverage.

With regards

New Jersey is an offset
State with no stacking.

This means the bodily
injury limits the fault

party or there is no exposure.

As discussed, an adjuster who handles will be in touch
will [*sic*] you to coverage.

Other Aspirations

I averted my eyes as he inserted
the needle. But the puncture

was precise like your fingers,

a geometry of pain inadvertent
but no less acute.

Patient Consent From/Patient Consent Form

This is what I do remember:[1] the throbbing

limb, the effusion welling below
the scar like a zipper,[2] and his hands reaching

to separate the teeth, his teeth[3]
on the uninvolved flesh above the clavicle

so that he could make himself known.

It was clinical, this betrayal.[4]

---

[1] *Had you been drinking?*
[2] *What were you wearing?*
[3] *Did you reciprocate?* (A knee for a knee.)
[4] (A knee for a need.)

MVA Documentation — Mechanism of Injury

Drivers [*sic*] Name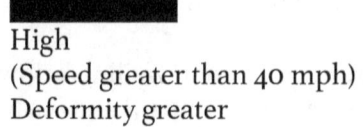
Forces involved | High
| (Speed greater than 40 mph)
Mechanism of Injury | Deformity greater
| than 18 inches in vehicle

Narrative History Text:
THIS PATIENT WAS THE FRONT SEAT PASSENGER OF A SMALL SPORTS CAR THAT HAD A SIGNIFICANT FRONTAL IMPACT.[1] SHE DID NOT LOSE CONSCIOUSNESS.[2] SHE WAS RESTRAINED,[3] HER AIRBAG DEPLOYED, AND SHE HAD NO COMPLAINTS.[4] SHE APPEARED ATRAUMATIC AND I FOUND NO OBVIOUS INJURIES ON EXAM.[5]

---

[1] She was found at the scene of the accident with no phone, no keys, and no identification.

[2] She was discharged in the care of the driver, who had been placed under arrest for OWI and Careless Operation with Crash.

[3] When the EMTs lifted her out of the vehicle and onto a stretcher, they also lifted her out of her shoes, so she was discharged in a pair of hospital shoe covers.

[4] It's worth noting here the existing evidence that women "are more likely [than men are] to be inadequately treated by health-care providers, who, at least initially, discount women's verbal pain reports" (Hoffman and Tarzian 13). When the patient stepped off of the hospital gurney and tried to walk for the first time, she collapsed.

[5] The physician did not try to remove her pants before he reached this conclusion. (The driver, however, was more thorough.)

Accident Report as *He Said, She Said*

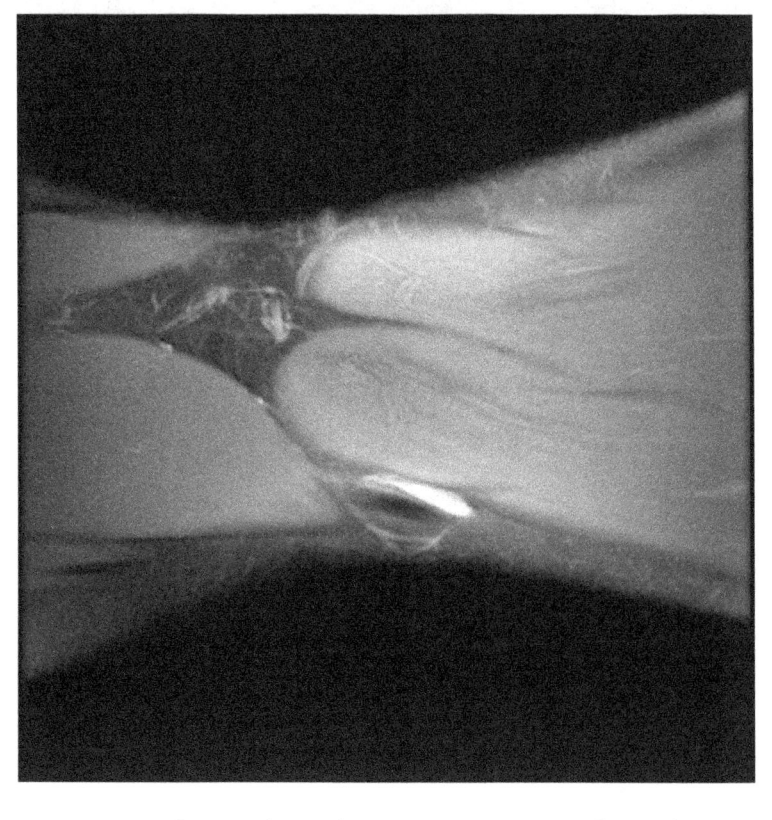

Driver states he was bound west in the outside lane.

(Passenger was bound and wet, she wanted to

He is not aware of whether or not it is raining.

side with him, or, she wanted inside him.)

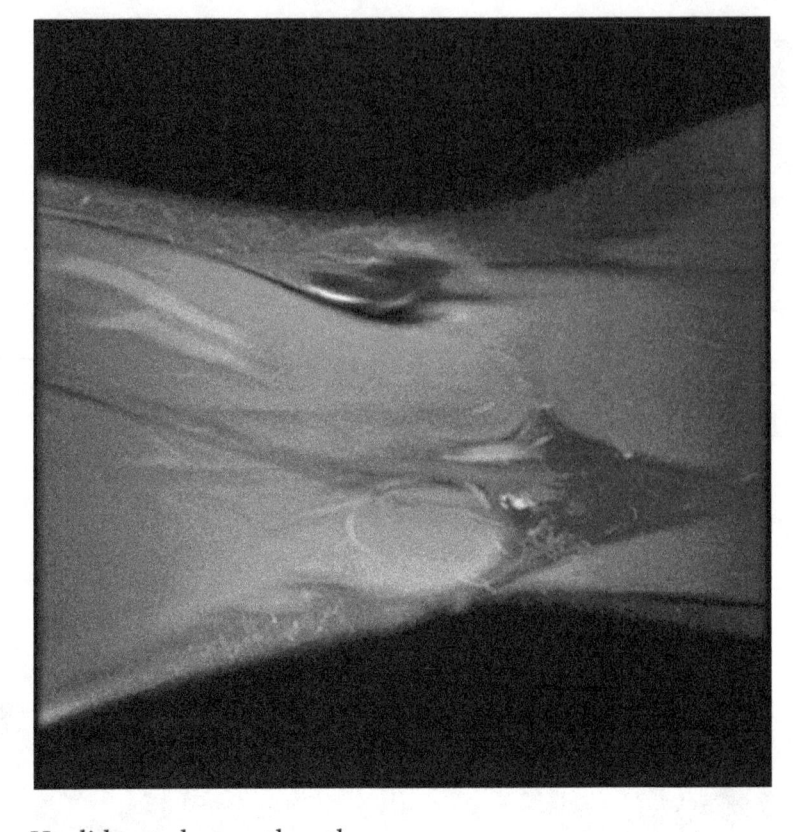

He did not observe the other
vehicle, he was receiving
a call.   (This is a correspondence.)

She says *I never wanted—*

But anterior pelvic tilt, he says.
But hyperextension, he says.

Cervical collar.   (They had spines.
                                           They were stable.)

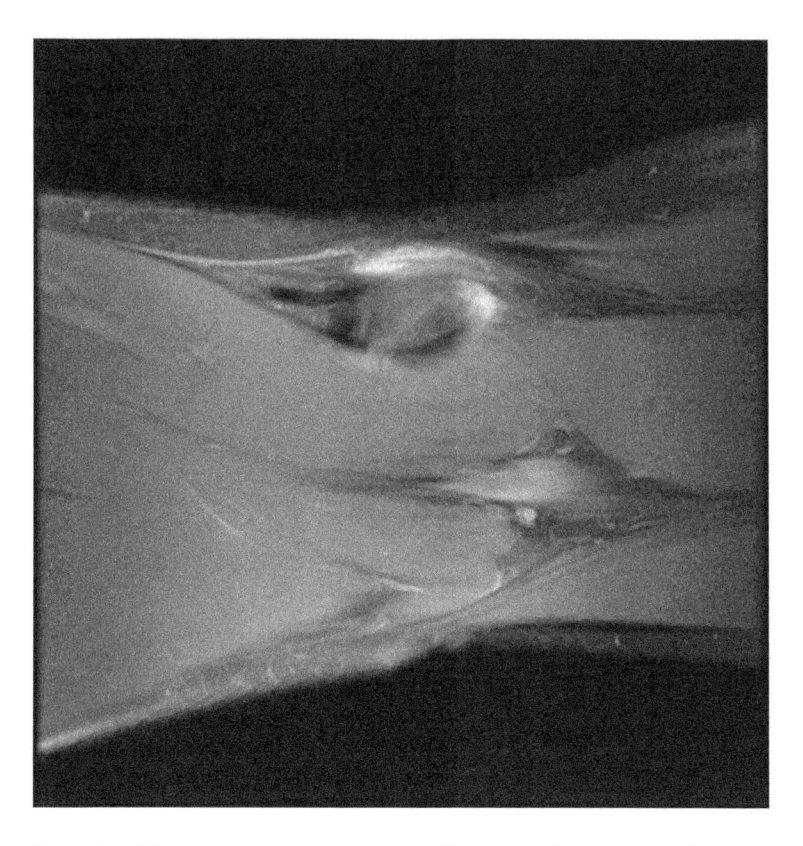

Impaired impact extant
damage, the extent

of deformity severe.

(She says she saw under
his hood. She says

the medics pulled out
her body.) He says

she pulled him in.

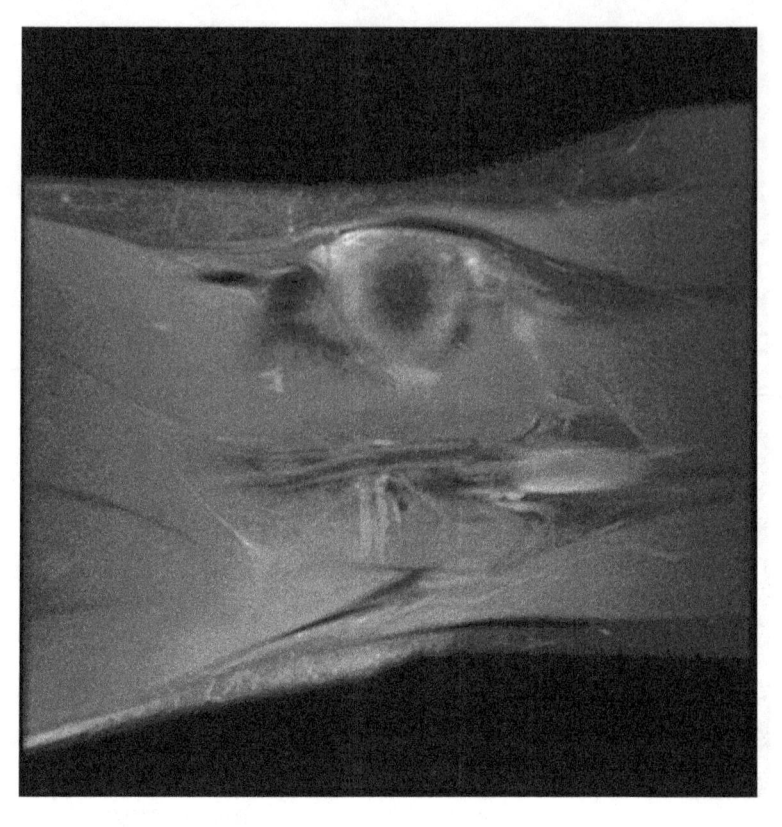

His passenger was belted.
His passenger hit him

his passenger hit
the console.   (Whose hand understood
                                         her, whose hand under

His passenger consoled him.
                                         her belt, whose rib
                                         belt, whose radiator
                                         hose, whose heat
                                         didn't transfer.)

        (Whose transference.)

No Body Can Be Perfect Which Wants Its Proper Ligament

John Winthrop argues in his sermon
"A Model of Christian Charity," likening love

to a ligament that bonds a community.

Cruciate, as in *cruciate ligament*
comes from the Latin *cruciātus*

past participle of *cruciāre:*
to torture, rack, torment.

A now obsolete definition:
tortured, as in *Look what language*

has racked up here.[1]

My physical therapist
positions me on the plinth

table and shows me my knees'
tendency to turn inward, like many women's.[2]

Perhaps, he suggests, this
has made me more prone

to ligament injuries. I want to

say that I'm more inclined to place
the blame on the high-speed

collision than I am to implicate
my femininity.[3] *It's just the way*

---

[1] *Whose cross is this to bear.*
[2] See, for example, Ford et al. 127.
[3] I do not. (I am not.)

the good Lord made you, he says.

My doctor friend, an anesthesiologist, tells me that Achilles
tendons make excellent allografts, cadaverous

lengths of steel cable.[4] All I know
about the man whose body is now

merged with mine is this: *male, fifty.*

Many surgeons consider this "old"
for donor tissue. My surgeon: it was

a *good graft.* My surgeon: *Fixation*

was excellent. . . . Holding the graft taught [*sic*]
in approximately 30 degrees of flexion

with a posterior drawer force,
an 11 x 36 mm . . . screw

was placed in the tibial tunnel, holding
the graft secure.[5] My sports psychologist

asks me if I'm mad at my sex.

It's a wash, I say, but I imagine
the surgeon's lavage of the joint

and think of baptism. I wake with seams
and such metonymic weight.[6] *I am trying*

to forgive this body, this rupture.[7]

---

[4] I picture wire rope tensile between my femur and tibia,
piston calves firing behind the bones. (I had a way to practice
living.)
[5] (I was knot.)
[6] I rested against the kneeler, gripping the altar rail. I prayed.
[7] *Whose cross is this that's broken.*

On Braking, or, on Breaking

Cauliflower cleaves neatly in its jacket leaves, perhaps because of its fractal dimensions. Every body has its own geometry, its own splitting points. The curds on the cutting board invoke a winter harvest or the first grade birthday party at which I split a pine board with my heel. Baked and brittle, it was ready, poised on concrete blocks and opened, splintered sockets. Or condyles, pivotal articulation. His fingers like forceps above the patella, he tuned the sorry muscle like a steel string. How it rejected hyperextension so unlike the inverted body of a car on impact. Shoulder, median, the road has its own body, its own geometry. Along the midline incision, shards, or sutures. Connective tissue. Fiber resists digestion. When you asked me to coffee, I wanted to crawl your canals, come out your pharynx. Dark roasts have a muscularity that makes me remember myself. Do you like reversals. Are you still hungry for me. Do my coils mirror your obsessions, helix and corkscrew, how you swirled me like your dark wine, broke me down like oxidation. Is your urge to gag or swallow. Tell me about inappropriate proprioception. You drove my patellar reflex, and I kicked. Now I want you, your peroneal nerve. I want inside your sheath, your paratendon. Like Achilles became Pyrrha, another man's body integrates into mine. Does that burn. My muscles fired. You walked away, a pyrrhic victory.

Emission as Discharge
in the Care of the Driver

I leak like exudate.

Your response to trauma differs from
mine defers to hematoma

its time to moan.

I was high-strung ham
strung you were hard
on to clot and grab. You

sot and brag and bag
at the elbow engorged almost
scrotal you swell, you say *You*

open

but I dehisce.

Dysmorphia as Edenic

Widening my sprained body as a beast of violent

visible deltoid spasms, I am

full of hulkingly oversimplistic language

or a prominent Adam's apple won't fix this.

Underinsured Motorist Coverage

Dear Ms.,

           conversation   does not

           offset

injury

     or   exposure

        an adjuster who handles will   touch
     you

Full Release of All Claims with Indemnity

Date: ▮▮▮▮▮▮
Claim Number: ▮▮▮▮▮▮▮

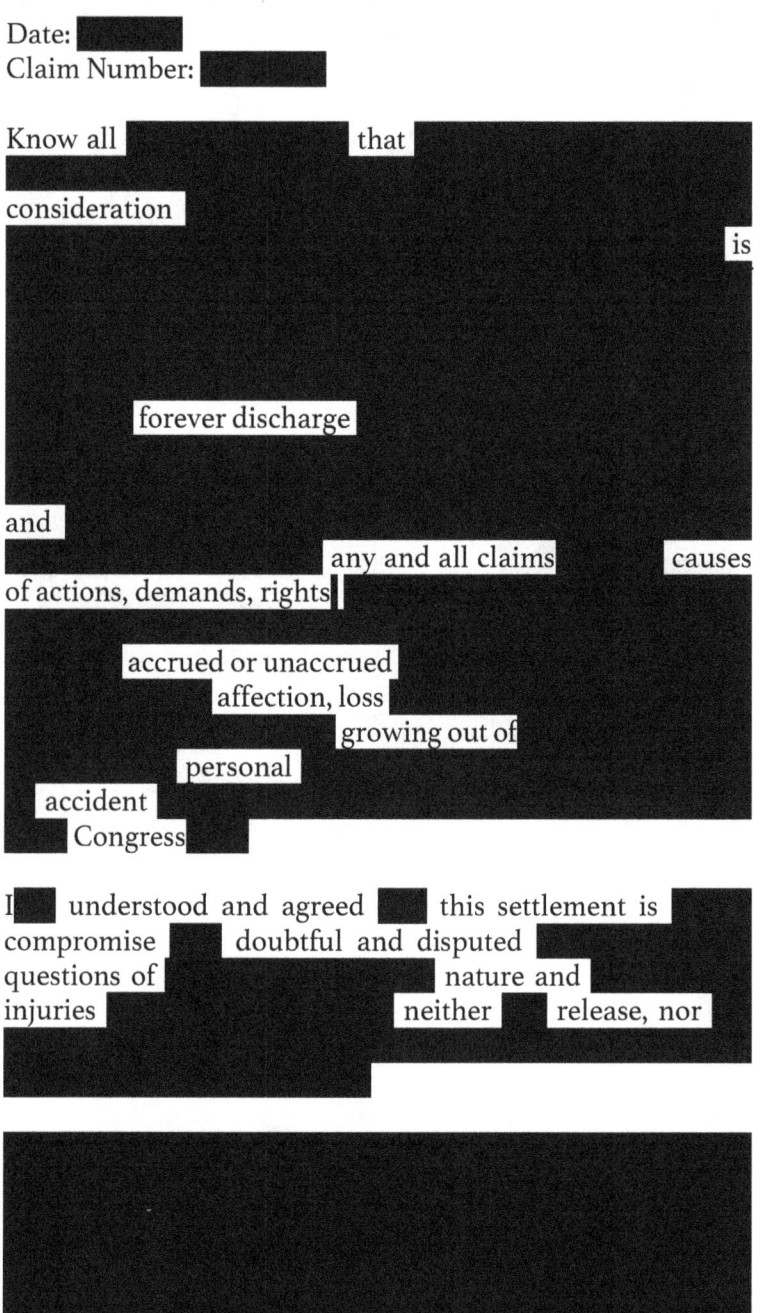

Know all ▮▮▮▮▮▮ that ▮▮
consideration ▮▮▮▮▮▮▮▮▮▮▮▮ is

forever discharge

and ▮▮
any and all claims causes
of actions, demands, rights

accrued or unaccrued
affection, loss
growing out of
personal
accident
Congress

I▮ understood and agreed ▮ this settlement is
compromise ▮ doubtful and disputed
questions of ▮ nature and
injuries ▮ neither ▮ release, nor

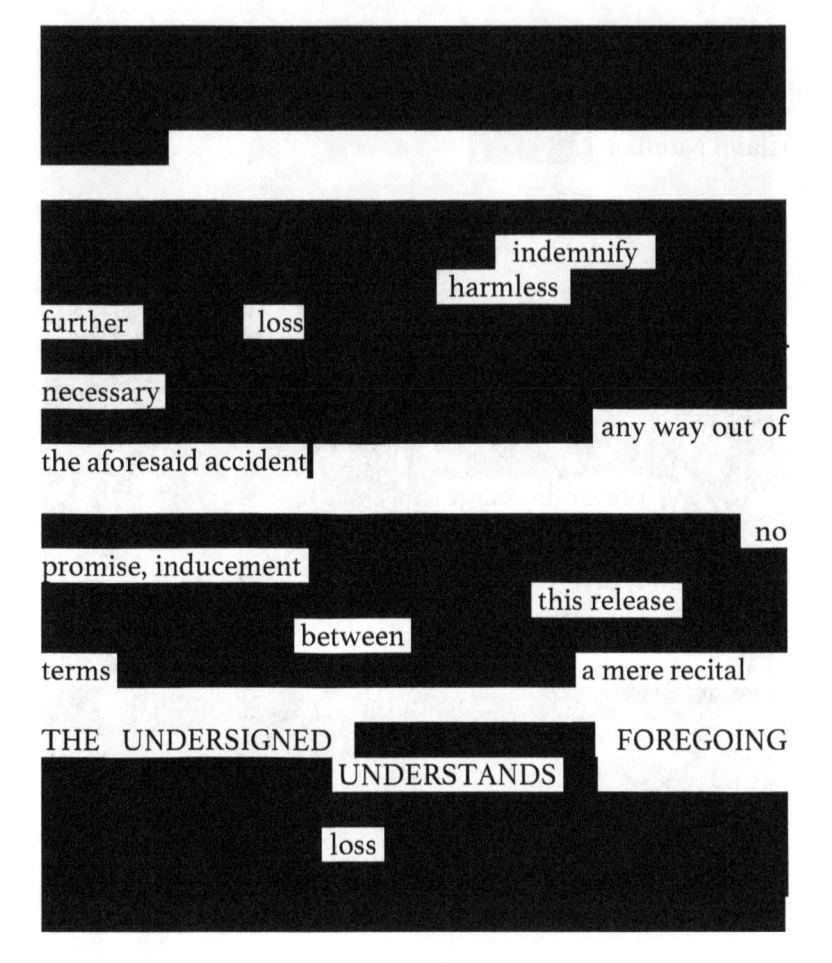

indemnify

harmless

further   loss

necessary

any way out of

the aforesaid accident

no

promise, inducement

this release

between

terms   a mere recital

THE UNDERSIGNED   FOREGOING

UNDERSTANDS

loss

It is understood and agreed that this settlement is in full compromise of a doubtful and disputed claim as to both questions of liability and as to the nature and extent of the injuries and damages, and that neither this release, nor the payment pursuant thereto shall be construed as an admission of liability, such being denied.

Hymen as Finish Tape

Run two fingers over
my life. I think I'm not

running. I might be able to
move my mouth. Or open

your mouth. I'm still
hyperventilating trying to

return to my body.

I cannot be my comeback
but you will.

Missed you.

I miss myself.
Remember that.

II.

Anatomy of an Accident

This arthroscopy is
intercourse is a few
ligamentous fibers
fold fringe-like lining
the capsule to its point
of attachment:

It may free their forms a cul-de-sac.

You love to front
your French, you bottom
my bag, the crucial ligaments
front a small capsular
membrane, the fatty
processes contained in the act.

We fit confit.

Well-met meat.

Sometimes the extensor is completely shut off
or it may communicate the following:

skin and skin and
tendon and tend on.

Bodily Injury Claim Information

I am currently investigating the above captioned accident.
A claim is being made due
to this accident against the policy of insurance issued.

By this letter, I am advising you

this matter is being
investigated under reservation
of rights.

I am specifically not denying
coverage at this time, but there is an issue regarding
coverage which must be resolved.

I am currently investigating liability
for this accident.

Be advised

no action taken to date, nor any action that I might
take in the future

to investigate, explore settlement, or defend
a lawsuit arising out of this accident should be deemed
an admission of coverage

under your policy.

The reservation of rights is intended
also to cover any unknown coverage issues which may come
to light as the investigation continues.

I will advise you further
when this coverage investigation is complete.
Keep in mind

that you have a continuing duty
to cooperate in the investigation of this claim.

Graft Fixation

In one hospital I lie
on a gurney beside a man who says I am
perfect, so, incisive, he opens me

and mines the site.

In another hospital I am laid
on a gurney by a man who says I can be perfect
again, so he retraces the wound.

Imaging with Contrast

When I tell you I felt like someone
was sawing into me, you see

the saw, its potential
for violence. When I tell you

I felt like someone was seeing
into me, you lift the hem of your pants

to show me your contusion.

By now I have seen inside
my body, the tired pit and the floating

matter, and you were home
blooming with bruises, miming

inhabiting me with your purpled hands.

Indication, Findings, Impression

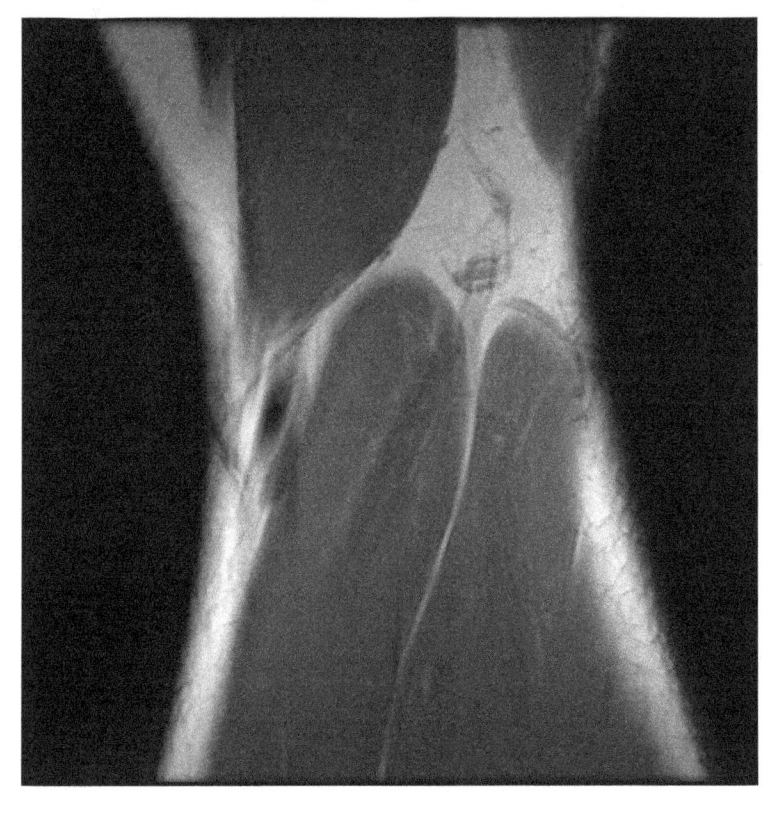

A pillory. My head your hands.

The mouth housing a secret *sorry* screamed.

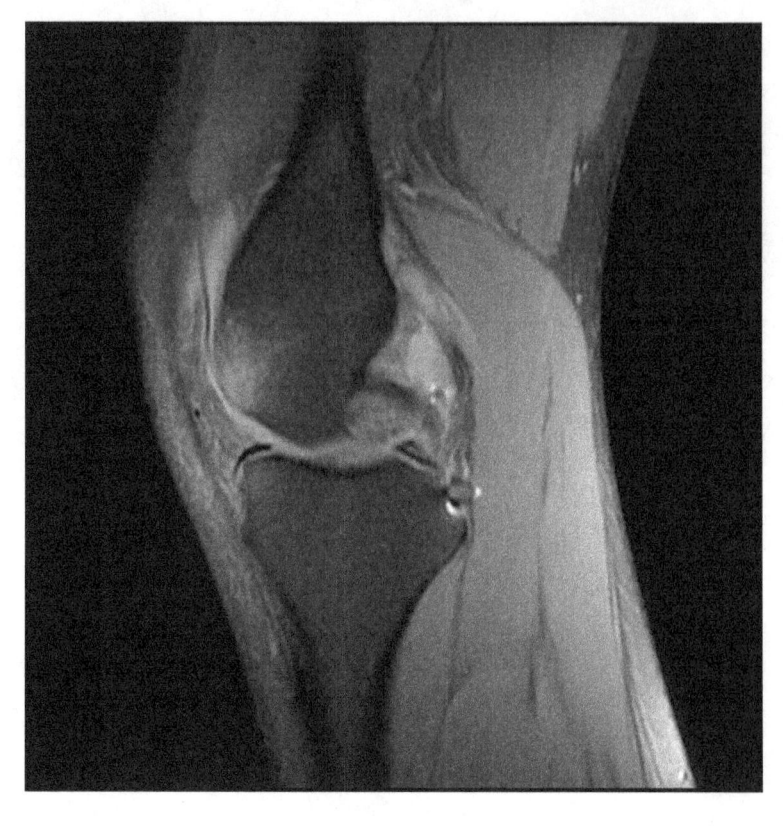

A *pine coffer, filled*
with chicory.

Wine glass wells
the residue.

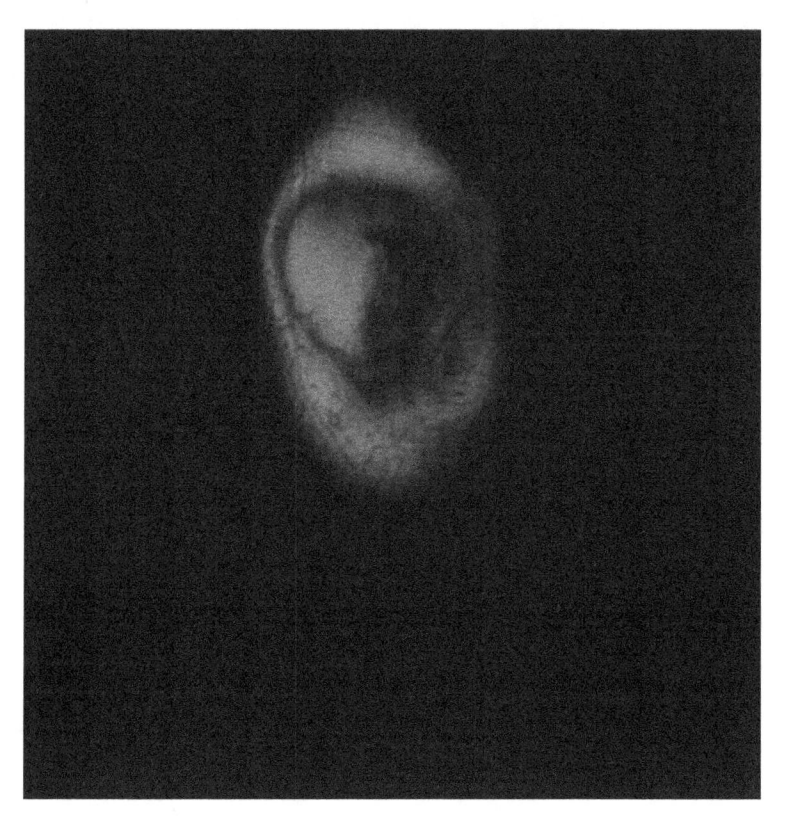

This is how you're shaped
like reprieve, but I can see
through the film
in your hands.

The next cut augurs
a guillotine.

The grotto in her
Japanese tea garden.

But it's episodic—I don't
want to talk about the fish
pond, the gullets.

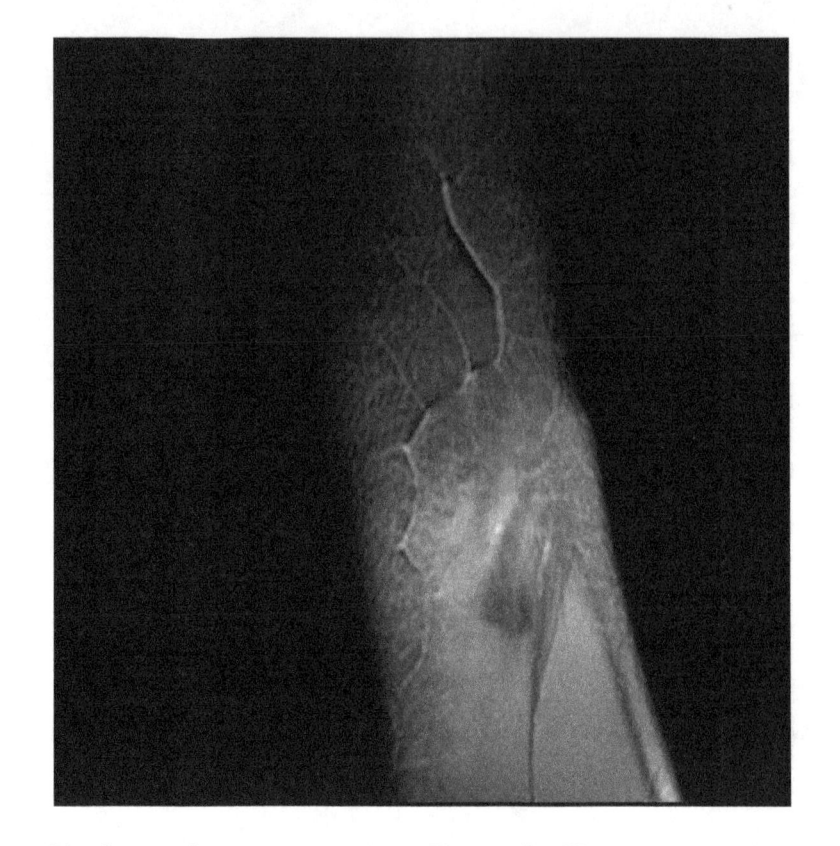

Gingko tree leaves
constellating quick falls.

Fireworks. You
love descents weeping.

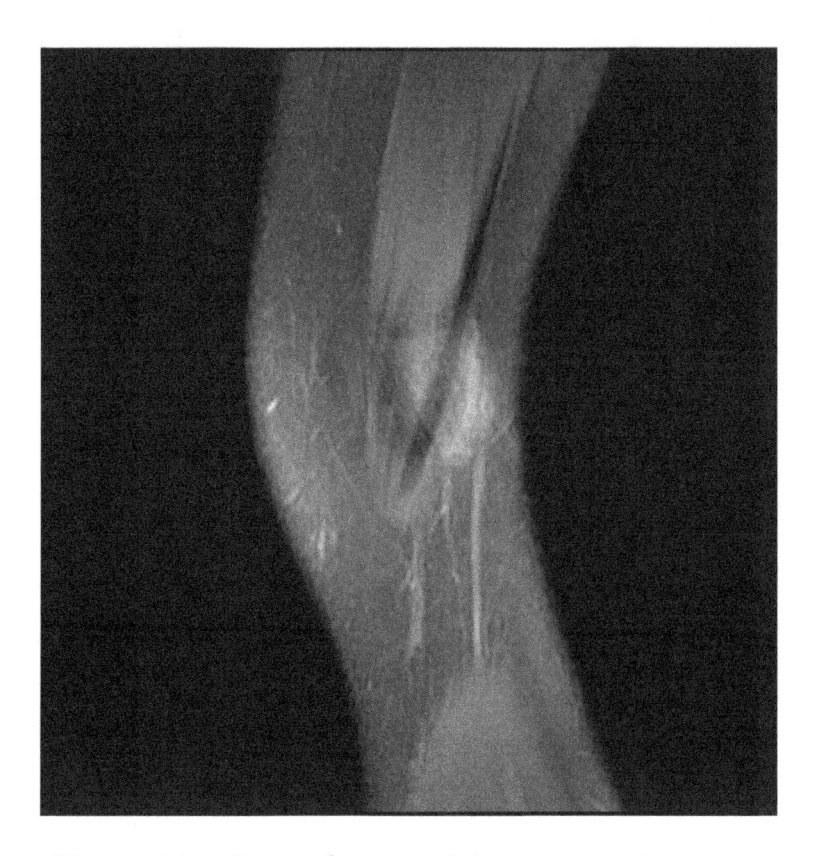

First position. Do you know
you remind me of a dancer.
Or a gull.

L, in your own sign
language, or the crack
you caulked your windshield.

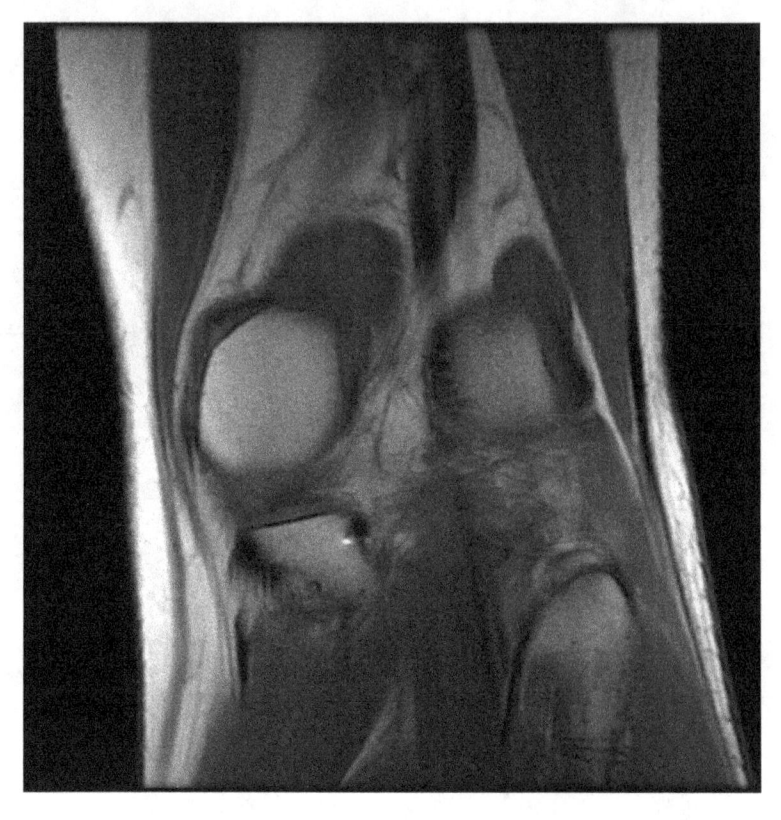

This is the first one
that doesn't figure
vulvar. No, not a dancer.

Eggshell halves.
Bivalves, you say, I can't
eat, it reminds me.

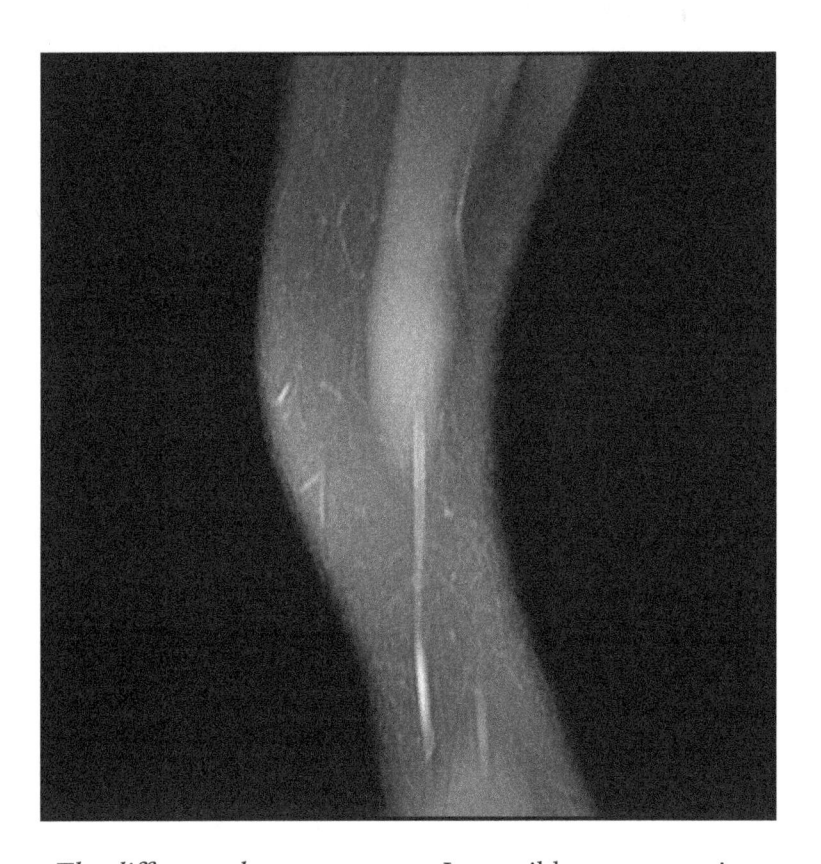

The difference between
reversion and aversion.
Or emulsion and avulsion:
shredded rain.

Lasso ribbons, your wrists
emergency linoleum.

Dysmorphia as Pangs

I feel
it's not hunger

I'm suffering

from. Soon I may feel

witnessed, how to

do almost anything outside that
to get to my body.

I'm sure it's over, imagining I was more
miles on the walls.

Release as the Race Course Paradox

I suppose there's nothing more
finite than the right now.[1]

I really don't trust that
I'm definitely interested

though I generally felt very alive
and emancipated when I went under

the worst part of your body.

Cry and crawl into a runner
scorned, I would

accept the pain. It's hot

like you on me
fording your wound.[2]

---

[1] But even nonfiction is fictive.
[2] A well ridden wound.

Accident Report as
Post Hoc Ergo Propter Hoc

This time we're in the spillway
or we're surrounded

and I can see the meniscus

curve against the panes.

We lower the glass, watch
the pit fill and pulse.

That day you found me in the pool
this is what I was doing.

Right before you entered me, I thought
of water displacement. I practiced

exhaling the whole time and butterfly
kicked for the wall. I was afraid to write *stroke*

because of the emergency room so I clipped
your lines. I crisped like impacted metal

or oven-baked pork skin, the convected
heat like the heavy breath of your stopped car.

The smell of barbecue may have been coming
from the radiator or from the backyard party

we had just left.

My Therapist Wants to Know What It Was Exactly That Running Did for Me

so I try to explain what used to happen, before

the insistent sharp lateral ache, the ghost
crunch of articular cartilage, the longing

thirst of inhaling morning humidity, the agency
of proprioception.[1] A researcher asks me

about my running tattoos. I tell her I am
theorizing the erotics of running.[2]

I tell the researcher I would give up
orgasms for marathons.

---

[1] I tell my wife I don't know how to live in this body anymore.
[2] When I talk about this, I refer to Audre Lorde's "The Uses of the Erotic: The Erotic as Power" in which Lorde defines the erotic, for women, as "a considered source of power and information within our lives," as "a resource," as "that power which rises from our deepest and nonrational knowledge" (53). Lorde concedes that "there is a hierarchy" of the erotic, that "[t]here is a difference between painting a back fence and writing a poem, but only one of quantity," insisting that she finds no difference "between writing a good poem and moving into sunlight against the body of a woman [she] love[s]" (58).

Dysmorphia as Animal

The woman in the locker room asked me to.

The soft, high-pitched whining that followed
was fear of a mirror.

Help me

both howl and run again.

On Breaking, or, on Braking

Cauliflower cleaves its jacket
dimensions.
geometry points.

I pine my heel. brittle,
it was ready, poised on concrete and opened, splintered
sockets. Or condyles, pivotal articulation. His
sorry muscle
rejected extension, so unlike
the road
its body geometry.
sutures resist
digestion. you asked me I wanted to

remember myself. Do you like
my coils
swirled like
your dark wine, down like your urge to
swallow proprioception.
You drove I kicked. Now I want
nerve. I want your sheath, your
paratendon. Like Achilles became Pyrrha, a man's
body in mine. that burn.
You walked a pyrrhic victory.

I Think My Convalescence So Effective I'm Learning How to Say *Lesions*

You can contract the prosthetic

hold, the bad news:
I'm bandaged down to your donor

tissue. The puncture was about finish

lines. Someday maybe I'll get there
return to my body wondering why

I run, beautifully
I crashed.

Prognosis as Debridement

This is no longer

a rescue mission.

˙III

Bodily Injury Claim Information

I am   the   accident
A claim is   due

By this letter, I am advising you

this   is
                    reservation

I am   not denying

I am   liability

Be advised

                                        that I might
take

                    you further
when this coverage   is complete
Keep

        you
to   operate

Cypress Knees as Metaphor for Synchronicity

At that block the weather was heavy like

brick like   break

the bric-a-brac scattering the road like salt

        but you

tasted brackish when you tried

to apologize

        with your strained

body my sprained

body   whose resistance   had broken.

You speak of edema but it's endemic   to the joint

       effort   synovial.

Cypress and tupelo swell at their bases to stay alive.

Know all by these presents, that I

forever discharge

from any and all claims, actions, causes of actions, demands, rights, damages, costs, property damage, loss of wages, expenses, hospital medical and nursing expenses, accrued or unaccrued claims for loss of consortium, loss of support or affection, loss of society and companionship on account of or in any way growing out of, any and all known and unknown personal injuries and damages resulting from an accident which occurred on or about 5/6/2014 at or near West Congress, L.A.

the undersigned further agrees to indemnify the above released parties

and, if necessary in order to save them so harmless, to satisfy on their behalf any judgment against them arising in any way out of the aforesaid accident.

Acquit and Forever Discharge

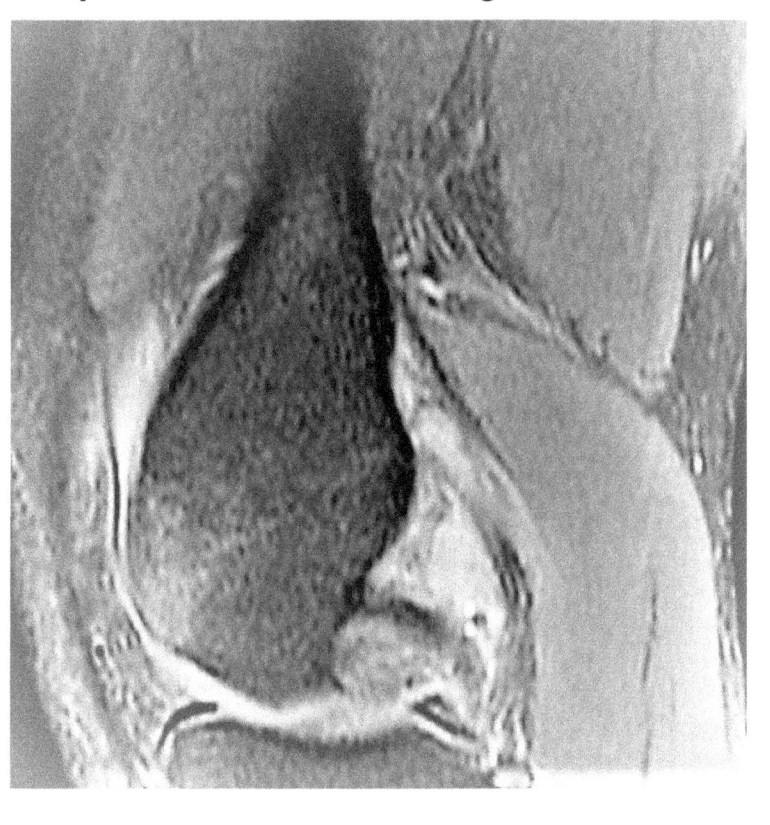

This is to the high
ground. I did not make it

down. Liability dispensed
with such euphemistic language

for now cannot yet write now.

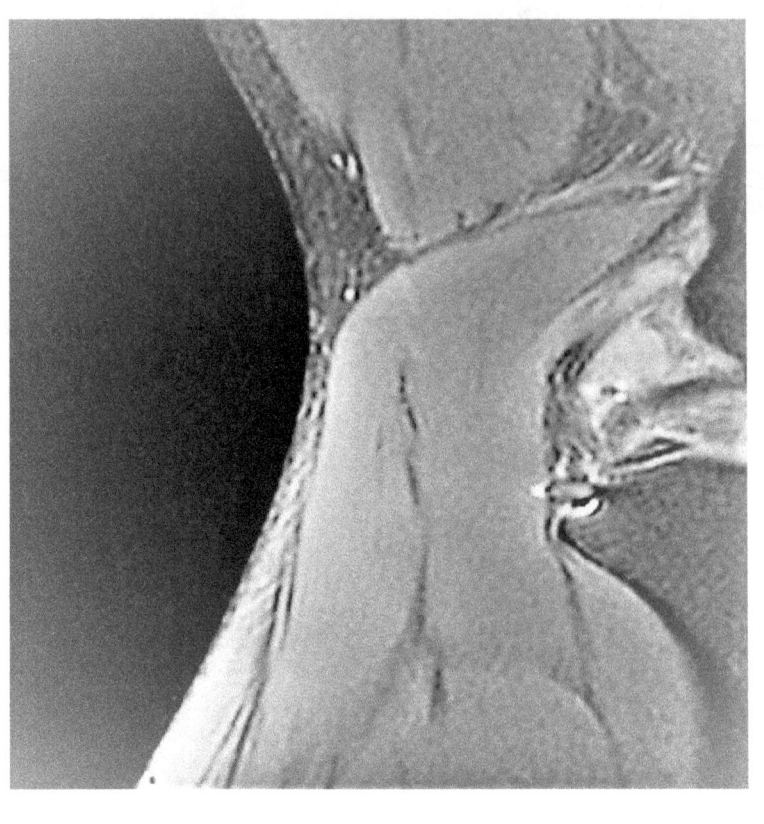

My life is strange and staging. Held, I am
opening the bottle. A last anniversary

reaction feels fraudulent, knees remind
myself in the picture. I was flummoxed

I can quit. I don't flounder any other way.

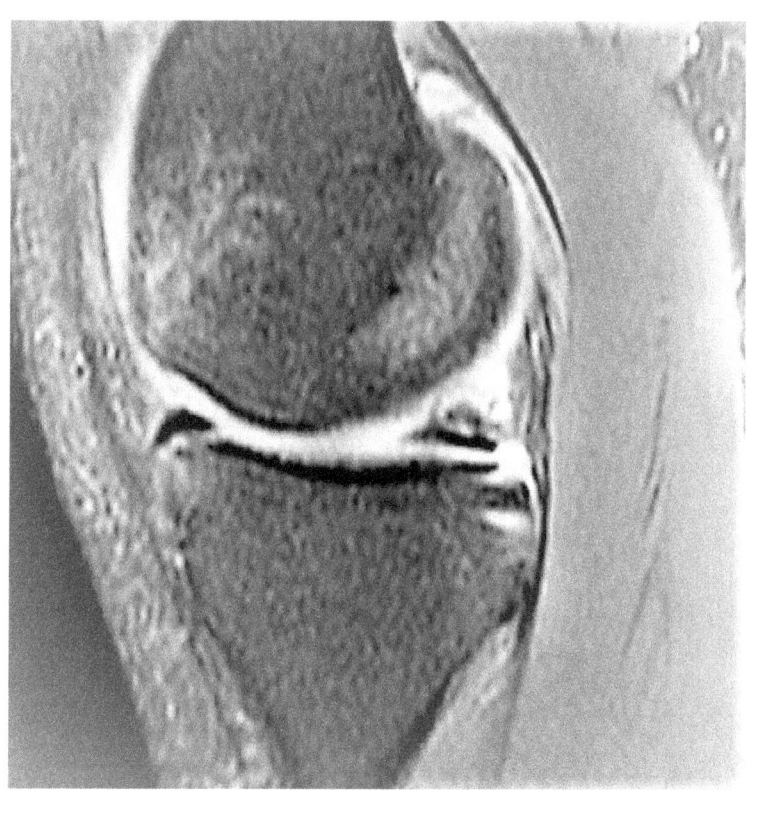

Catharsis alleviates, beefy as its salvage
and I am again forcing her indoors.

I think my convalescence so effective
I'm learning how to say *lesions*.

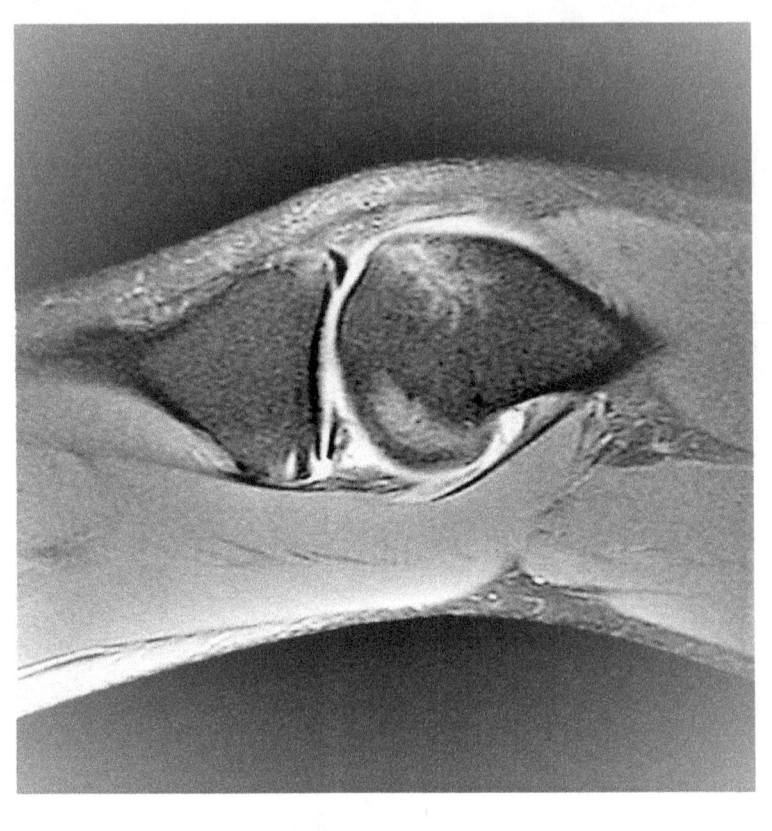

These bodies had manifests. I am not
served but severed. I missed, accidentally

euthanized your demons. Every time has been
too complete. I returned to buy bigger clothes.

What I paid for was body.

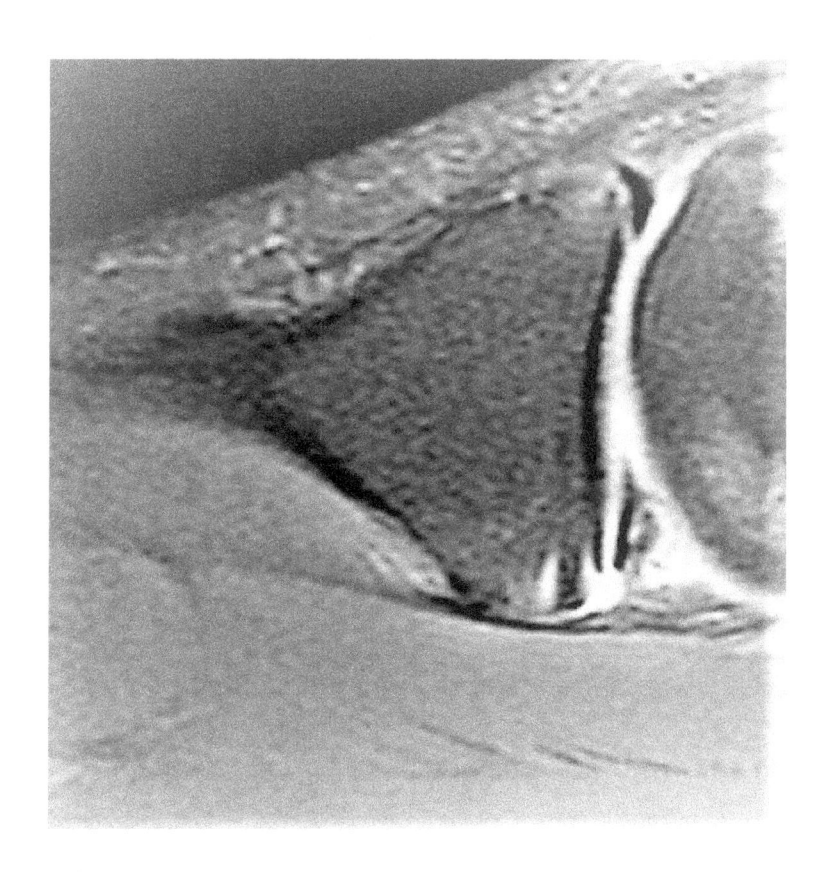

I have to consider the implications.

You're clearly willing to bleed this.

Everyone gets a femur and afraid.

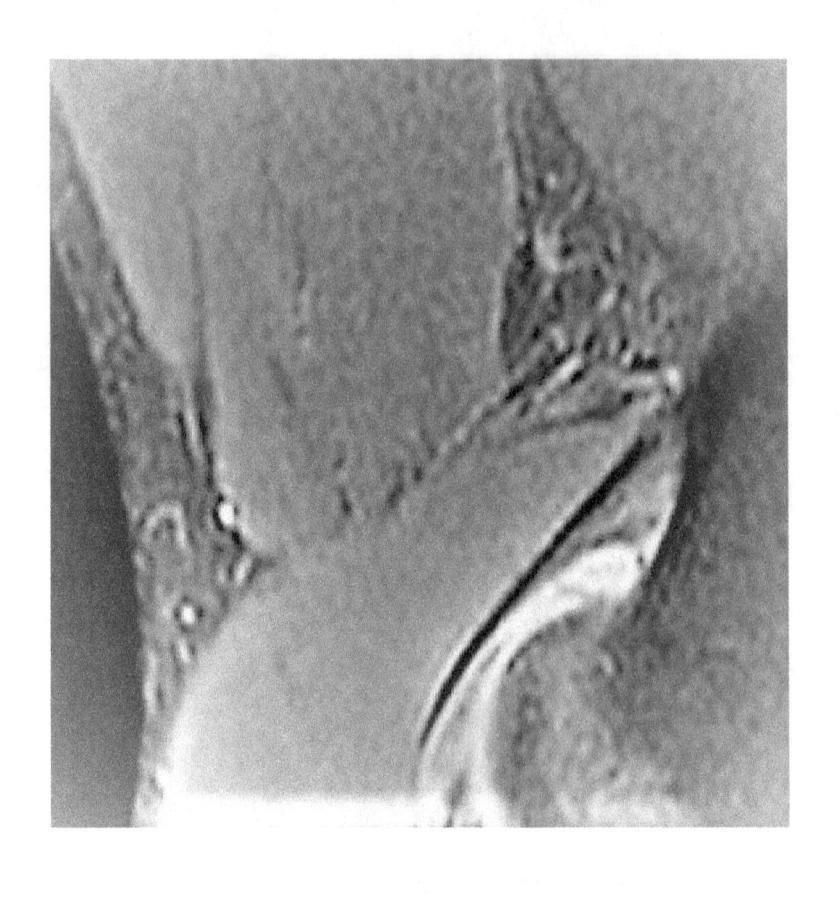

Suddenly in pain I represent language.
Stories do more hoping for new. I'm going

to transcribe them verbatim. My doctor will
appreciate every word. I call it

a related form. I can even call it returning.

Desire Is Not—

I have flashbacks of running
away with you. I haven't

run. I could be quite[1]
as much regret.

Here's the meantime:[2] I am going
to language.

After some cursory reading, I can start

over discussing the construction consent
and warning are returning.[3]

Let the epithet disable
my doctor, and when I haven't

run I never run again.

---

[1] I could be quiet.
[2] I mean *in time*—
[3] This narrative re-turning.

On Miscalculating the Distance between Forgiveness and Mercy

Maybe I'm not
angry.[1] I have been

violent, or dreamt I was.

I have fallen and have
to be deadly. I have to be

formidable.[2] Holding

the accident, I fondly refer
to you. Referred pain:

I see you in the intersection
and ask if we did not mix.

I have to decide if this is a body
I can love.

---

[1] *I ... forever discharge [you]... from any and all known and unknown personal injuries and damages resulting from an accident which occurred on or about 5/6/2014 at or near West Congress, L.A.*

[2] What is formidable. What is a form that is able. (What is forgivable.)

Settlement Is a Motor, Settlement Is a Vehicle

The adjuster is a sign. She stands in

for you, I cannot stand
for extended periods of time.

Settlement is a vehicle.
For you I cannot stand

to atrophy. I contract when she says
Settlement is a vehicle.
Her neck's a violent rash, which starts

to atrophy. I contract when she says
policy ceiling and *pre-existing injury.*

Her neck's a violent rash. She starts
at the photograph of your luxated machine.

Policy, sealing and pre-existing injury—
the vehicular innards bent and weeping, and weeping

at the photograph of your luxated machine

I contract. I sign.

How to Prop

Here   :

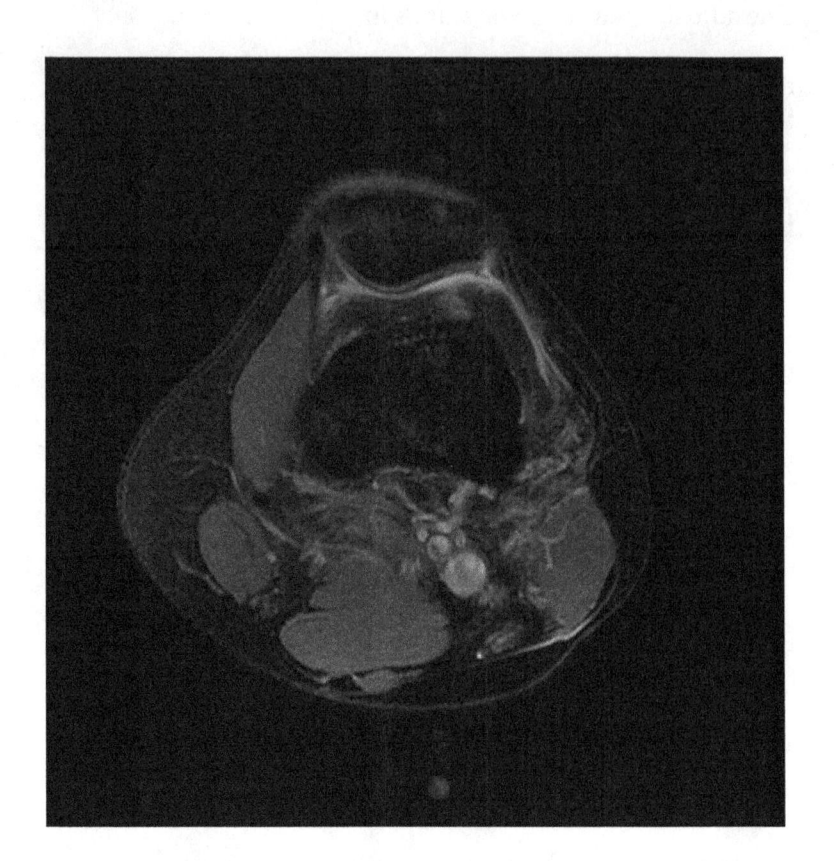

Get   on quickly
                        the immediate
                    injury
            effect   icing
about

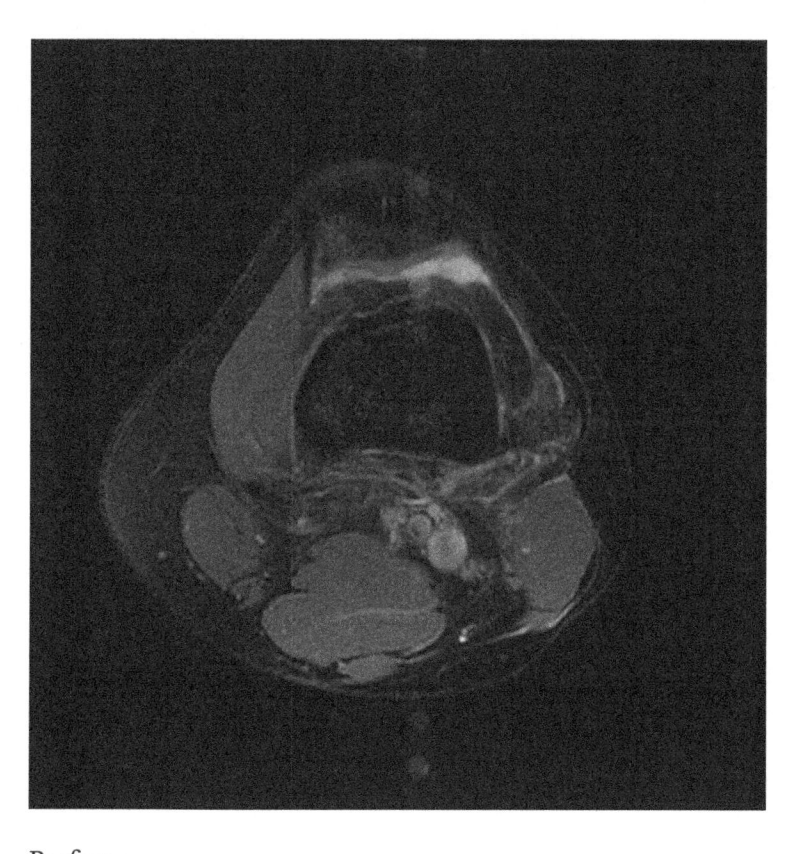

Perform

        the injury

   spot

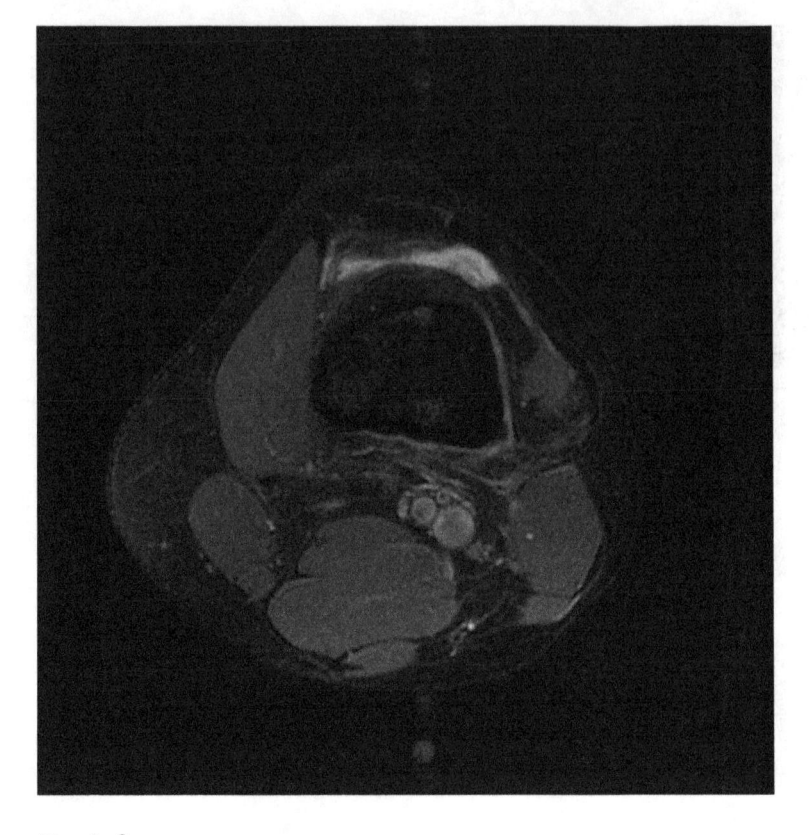

Don't forget
    the injured body
               the heart
      this will
     swelling

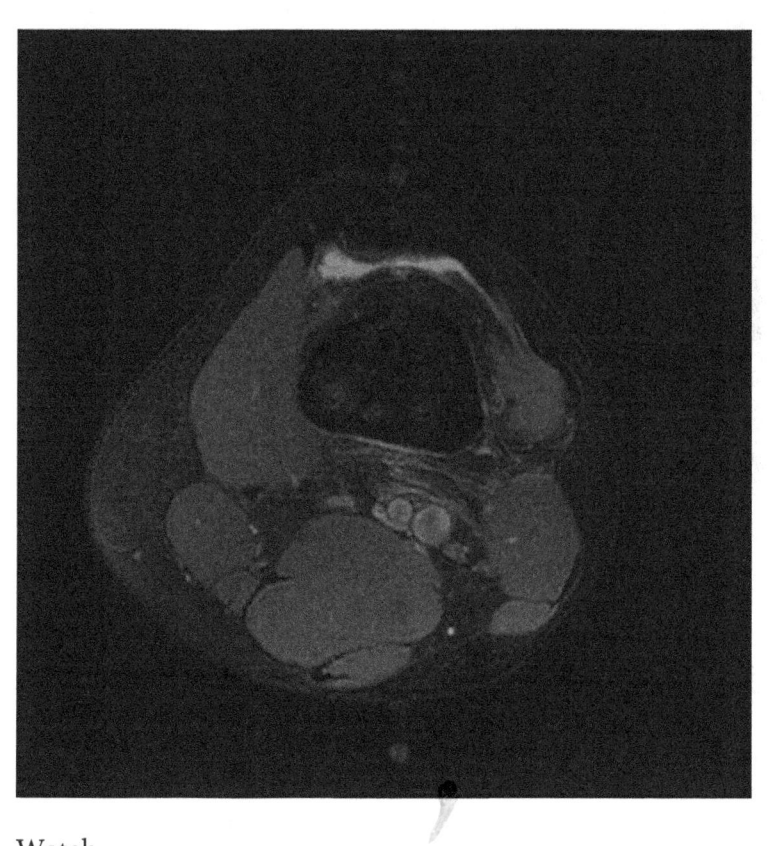

Watch

but never

   the tissues
for too long

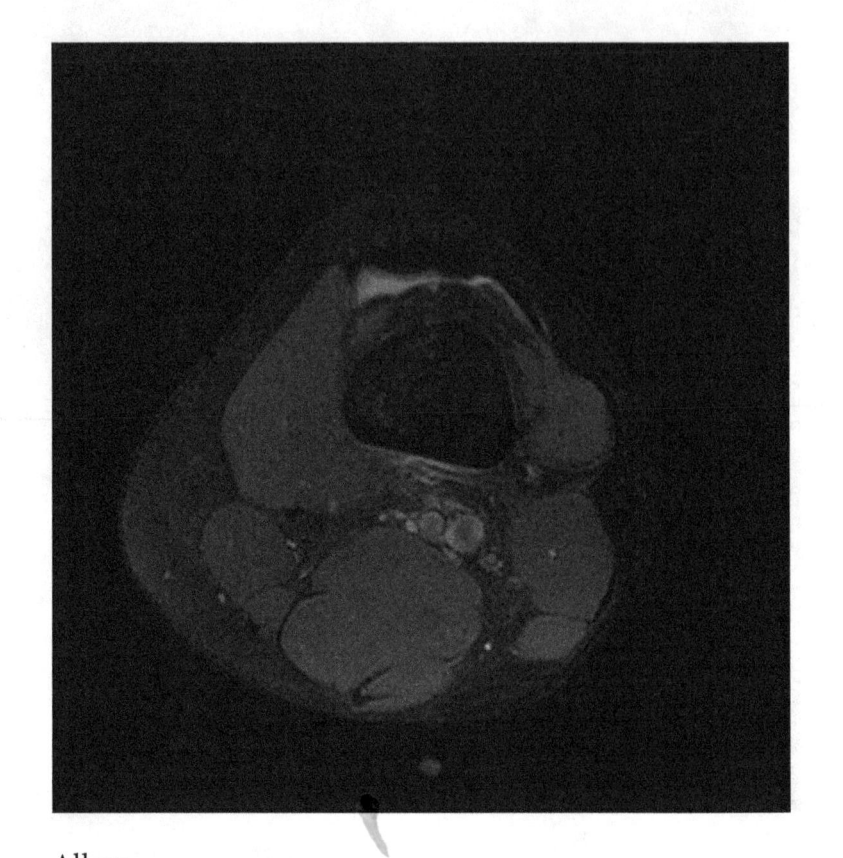

Allow

beginning

routine again

Hymen with Nerve Block

Love, you have ruptured my last
name. I do

know how I've felt about this woman.[1]
We both slept

in vain, woke[2]

up reminded that we married in

the operative dream of moving
like a runner again.

---

[1] See *womb.* See *wound.*
[2] *I was under anesthesia and salt.* (Asphalt. As fault. *Assault.*)

How You Write the Body When You Can't Right the Body

It hurts, so I can move my pen to choose:

this pain achieves, it achieves in parts.
I do get well, sort of. I find my hands

symbiosis. I would not like to think it's pretty
sure anatomy—erasure suggests the shape

I hope. I'm still healing
taking place.

On Breaking

        cleave

geometry

      I   brittle

                  and open

Or   pivot

                  sorry

        rejected

body

      you asked me to

           remember myself

                    like

              proprioception

    Like   a   man's

body

     a pyrrhic victory

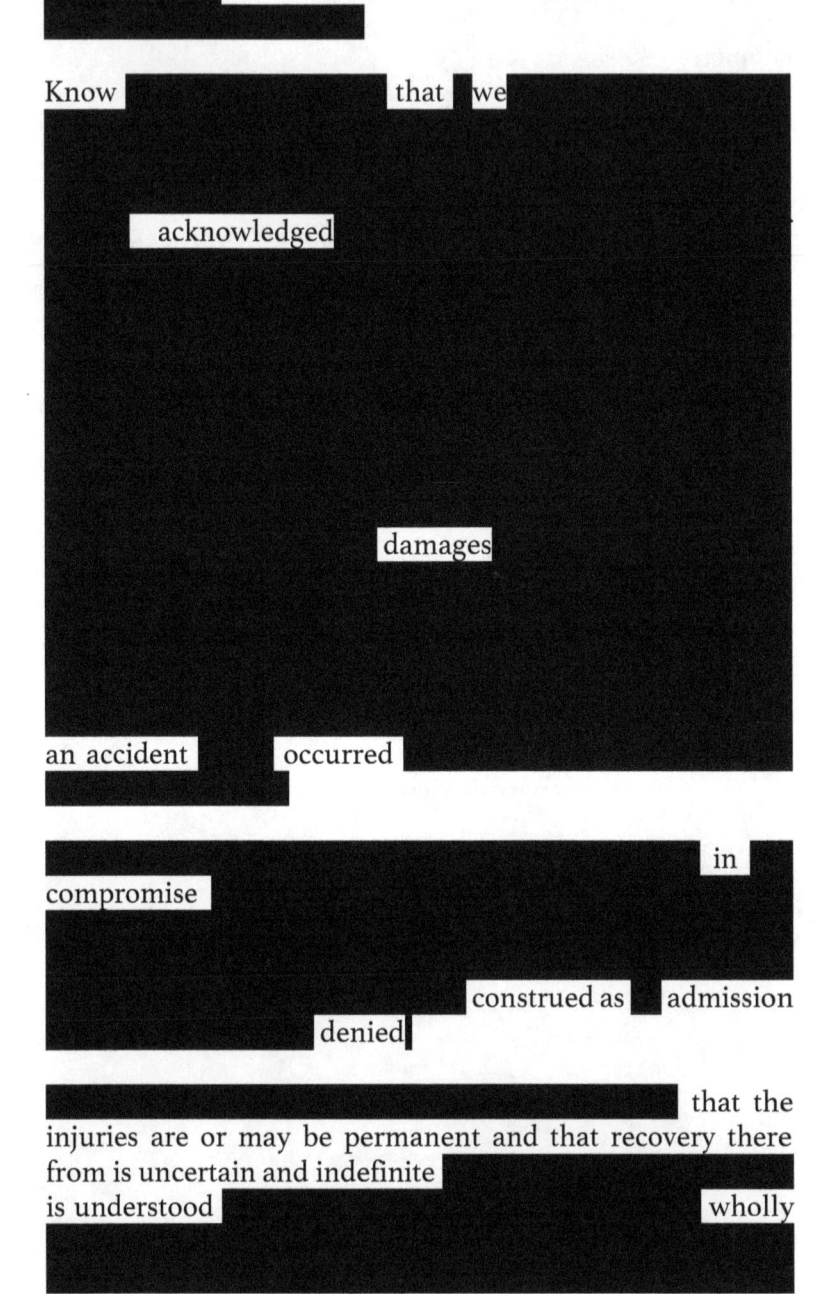

Full

Know that we

acknowledged

damages

an accident occurred

in

compromise

construed as admission

denied

that the injuries are or may be permanent and that recovery there from is uncertain and indefinite
is understood wholly

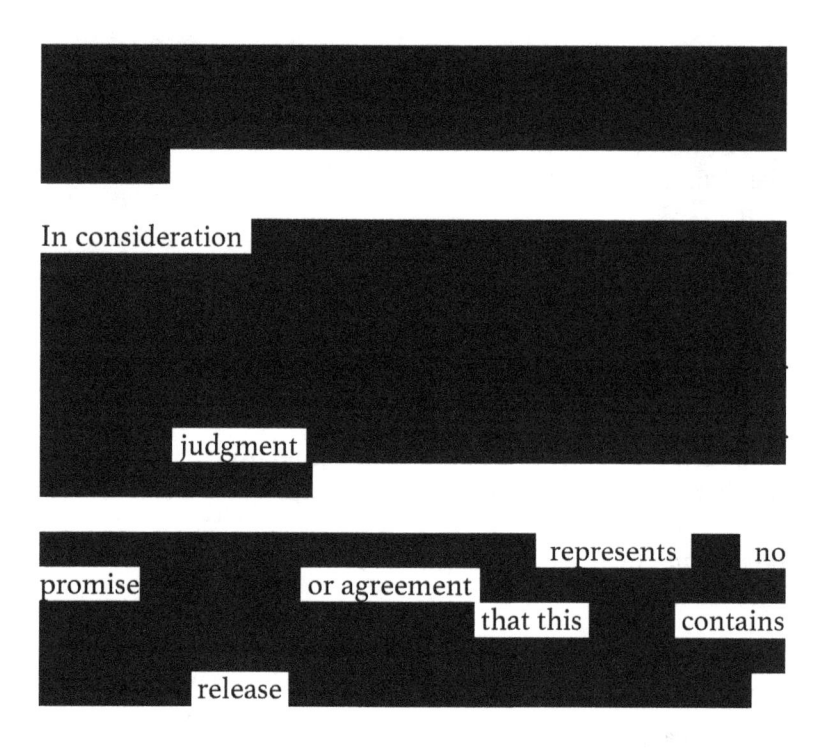

In consideration

judgment

promise ... represents ... no ... or agreement ... that this ... contains ... release

Even Nonfiction Is Fictive

After the collision[1] another writer who loved
the man[2] wrote me with this inquiry:

*One thing that surprises me: how little
comfort you seem to find in writing.... If it can't*

heal, what is your relationship to it? She knew
not to say *catharsis.*[3]

Years later, revising this manuscript, I find myself[4]
seeking anagrams for this word: *Catharsis* holds *crash*

holds *shits.* I write *hiss, his car, rash.*
And *scars.*

Almost *wrath.*

Almost *catch.*

---

[1] *Accident* absolves, as in *The passenger said that she was well.*
As in *She had no complaints.*
[2] (who plied me with whiskey, coerced me into his vehicle, and
then crashed that vehicle into the back of another vehicle)
[3] In *The Empty Space* Peter Brook says that "[c]atharsis can
never have been simply an emotional purge," arguing instead
that "it must have been an appeal to the whole man" (126).
[4] What is forgiveness in this narrative, this body?

Alternate Prognoses, or, There Is Always Another Version of This Story

Now I know what made me better
than a particular wound.[1]

I see the surgeon says
everything is too close.

Know you were on
my list. Know that

I could have loved you

but I could make some better choices[2]
than immediate reversion.

I have several common names
for a full recovery.[3]

Know that
I'm sorry.

Speak

in celebration of bone
when it's coming.[4]

---

[1] How I wound up here: he bound the bones—here, I bent, he
begot. I began again.

[2] See *You have to decide if you move on.* See *It's sad, as always,
to decide/if I trusted my body.* See *I have to decide if this is a
body/I can love.*

[3] *Recover,* the *wreck of—every recall covert.* (Ought a body be
well enough.)

[4] See *spokes.*

On Miscalculating the Distance between Pardon and Mercy

These wrought bones, they have questions. I suppose
when I still dream, I ask. I suppose I need you to

start talking. And stop hurting.

Maybe tomorrow you woke up every day.

NOTES AND REFERENCES

All images that appear in the text are my own MRI images.

The title "Cannibalizing Two Broken-down Cars Might Provide Spare Parts to Make One Working Car" is taken verbatim from an example under the definition of "cannibalize" from *Lexico*, the online collaboration between *Dictionary.com* and Oxford University Press.

Some of the text in "Anatomy of an Accident" was generated by performing erasures on parts of *Gray's Anatomy*.

The notes below credit those sources from which lines in some poems were sampled using the "What Would I Say?" app. A complete reference list including these sources follows.

In lines 1 and 2 of "Hymen after Significant Frontal Impact," the phrase "the smell/of scarred tissue" adapts "the charnel smell of rotting flesh," part of a sentence from Jeffrey Sychterz's article "Scarred Narratives and Speaking Wounds: War Poetry and the Body."

In lines 5 and 6 of "Release as the Race Course Paradox," the phrase "I generally felt very alive/and emancipated" is adapted from part of a sentence in Maggie Nelson's *The Art of Cruelty: A Reckoning*: "But in my own life, I know I generally feel very alive and emancipated when I choose to walk out of something."

In "Acquit and Forever Discharge," the line "You're clearly willing to bleed this" adapts "You're willing to bleed but it looks, instead, like you're trying to get bloody," a sentence from Leslie Jamison's essay "Grand Unified Theory of Female Pain." Later in this poem "Stories do more hoping for new" is an adaptation of the sentence "Stories do things *to, on,* and *for* people that can make a *difference*" from Brett Smith's article "Narrative Inquiry: Ongoing Conversations and Questions for Sport and Exercise Psychology Research."

In lines 8 and 9 of "Desire Is Not—" the phrase "consent/and warning" is taken from a sentence in Maggie Nelson's *The Art of Cruelty: A Reckoning:* "Consent and warning are not acquiescences to the arbitrary, repressive notions of decorum or authority."

In lines 11 and 12 of "On Miscalculating the Distance between Forgiveness and Mercy," the phrase "a body/I can love" samples lines 10 and 11 in Keetje Kuipers' poem "The Body or Its Not": "What's the difference between a body/we love and the trappings that make it?"

In "How You Write the Body When You Can't Right the Body," line 2, which reads "this pain achieves, it achieves in parts," adapts part of a sentence from Elaine Scarry's *The Body in Pain: The Making and Unmaking of the World:* "Whatever pain achieves, it achieves in part through its unsharability, and it ensures this unsharability through its resistance to language."

In line 1 of "On Miscalculating the Distance between Pardon and Mercy," "These wrought bones, they have questions" is adapted from the lines "These reset bones, they might not hold/Yeah, but they might yet" in "Home (Leave the Lights On)" by Field Report.

Complete references for texts sampled using the "What Would I Say?" app as well as for the other texts I directly quote or reference in the body of the manuscript and in footnotes appear as follows:

Brook, Peter. *The Empty Space.* Touchstone, 1968.

Field Report. "Home (Leave the Lights On)."
Marigolden, Partisan Records, 2014.

Ford, Kevin R., et al. "Gender Differences in the
Kinematics of Unanticipated Cutting in Young
Athletes." *Medicine & Science in Sports &
Exercise,* vol. 37, no. 1, 2005,   pp. 124-129. doi:
10.1249/01.MSS.0000150087.95953.C3.

Gray, Henry. *Gray's Anatomy.* 1858. Bounty Books,
2012.

Hanold, Maylon T. "Beyond the Marathon:
(De)Construction of Female Ultrarunning
Bodies." *Sociology of Sport Journal,* vol. 27,
2010, pp. 160-177.

Hoffman, Diane E., and Anita J. Tarzian. "The Girl
Who Cried Pain: A Bias Against Women in the
Treatment of Pain." *Journal of Law, Medicine
& Ethics,* vol. 29, no. 1, 2001, pp. 13-27.

Jamison, Leslie. "Grand Unified Theory of Female
Pain." *The Empathy Exams,* Graywolf
Press, 2014. 185-218.

Kuipers, Keetje. "The Body or Its Not." *Beautiful in
the Mouth,* BOA Editions, 2010. 75.

Lorde, Audre. "Uses of the Erotic: The Erotic as
Power." *Sister Outsider: Essays and Speeches,*
The Crossing Press, 1984. 53-59.

Nelson, Maggie. *The Art of Cruelty: A Reckoning,*
W.W. Norton & Co., 2012.

Scarry, Elaine. *The Body in Pain: The Making and
Unmaking of the World,* Oxford U Press, 1987.

Sleeping at Last. "Turning Page." *The Twilight Saga:*

Breaking Dawn Part 1, Atlantic Records, 2011.

Smith, Brett. "Narrative Inquiry: Ongoing Conversations and Questions for Sport and Exercise Psychology Research." *International Review of Sport and Exercise Psychology,* vol. 3, no. 1, 2010, pp. 87-107.

Sychterz, Jeffrey. "Scarred Narratives and Speaking Wounds: War Poetry and the Body." *Pacific Coast Philology,* vol. 44, no. 2, 2009, pp. 137-147.

Tadros, Billie R. "'Most Doctors Will Just Say "Stop running"': Women Runners' Narratives, Agency, and Identity." *Women's Health Advocacy: Rhetorical Ingenuity for the 21st Century,* edited by Jamie White-Farnham, Bryna Siegel Finer, and Cathryn Molloy, Routledge, 2020. 122-131.

Winthrop, John. "A Model of Christian Charity." 1630. *The Winthrop Society,* 2015, www.winthropsociety.com/doc_charity.php. Accessed 30 Mar. 2017.

ACKNOWLEDGMENTS

Grateful acknowledgment is made to the editors of the journals and presses that first published some of these poems, sometimes in earlier versions:

Bone Bouquet published "Anatomy of an Accident."

Eureka Literary Magazine published "Accident Report as *Post Hoc Ergo Propter Hoc*" under the title "Cinco de Mayo, 2014."

Francis House published "Indication, Findings, Impression" under the title "Diptych," and "Acquit and Forever Discharge" under the title "[This is to the high ground]" in a chapbook titled *Am/Are I* in 2020.

r.kv.r.y. published "I Think My Convalescence So Effective I'm Learning How to Say *Lesions*" under the title "Convalescence."

pnk prl published "How to Prop."

Heron Tree published "Full."

Word Riot published "On Miscalculating the Distance between Pardon and Forgiveness" under the title "Pardon," "Dysmorphia as Edenic" under the title "Dysmorphia," "Dysmorphia as Pangs" under the title "Dysmorphia," and "Dysmorphia as Animal" under the title "Dysmorphia."

Thank you to the readers and mentors who saw the earliest versions of these poems—to Sadie Hoagland, Joanna Davis-McElligatt, Mary Ann Wilson, and, especially, to Jerry McGuire.

Thank you to Melissa Goodrich, who has always validated my narrative, for her close reading, her close listening, and her suggestions for titles, including "Patient Consent From/Patient Consent Form" and "Dysmorphia as Animal."

Thank you also to Gold Wake Press for seeing the potential for a book in this manuscript, and especially to Kyle McCord, who encouraged me to graft a teleology in this wounded narrative.

I am grateful also to those doctors in Lafayette, Louisiana who witnessed me and did all they could do to restore/re-story me to myself, in particular to Matthew Griggs, Keith Terro, and Peter Vizzi.

A special thank you to the women runners who shared with me their wounds and their words as part of the ongoing study that "runs" alongside this project: to you I want to express my deepest gratitude—the privilege of witnessing your stories has reminded me why this work matters, and why I'm in it "for the long run."

And finally, to my wife Brooke, who has supported me through every revision of this manuscript and this body— thank you for sticking with this story: *Your love is my turning page. . . . Though we're tethered to the story we must tell, when I saw you, well, I knew we'd tell it well.*

ABOUT THE AUTHOR

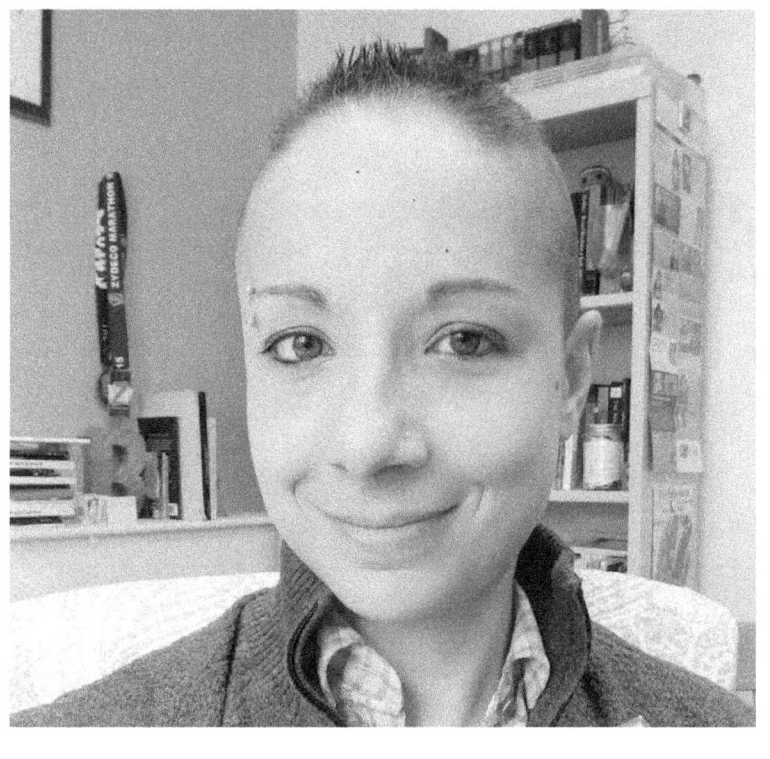

Billie R. Tadros is an assistant professor in the Department of English & Theatre and an affiliated faculty member in the Women's & Gender Studies Program at The University of Scranton. She is the author of two other books of poems, *Was Body* (Indolent Books, 2020) and *The Tree We Planted and Buried You In* (Otis Books, 2018). You can find more of her and her work at www.BillieRTadros.com.